77 Hair Loss Preventing Meal and Juice Recipes:

Using Hair Growing Vitamins and Minerals to Give Your Body the Tools It Needs

By

Joe Correa CSN

COPYRIGHT

ACKNOWLEDGEMENTS

This book is dedicated to my friends and family that have had mild or serious illnesses so that you may find a solution and make the necessary changes in your life.

77 Hair Loss Preventing Meal and Juice Recipes:

Using Hair Growing Vitamins and Minerals to Give Your Body the Tools It Needs

By

Joe Correa CSN

CONTENTS

ABOUT THE AUTHOR

After years of Research, I honestly believe in the positive effects that proper nutrition can have over the body and mind. My knowledge and experience has helped me live healthier throughout the years and which I have shared with family and friends. The more you know about eating and drinking healthier, the sooner you will want to change your life and eating habits.

Nutrition is a key part in the process of being healthy and living longer so get started today. The first step is the most important and the most significant.

INTRODUCTION

77 Hair Loss Preventing Meal and Juice Recipes: Using Hair Growing Vitamins and Minerals to Give Your Body the Tools It Needs

By Joe Correa CSN

Bright, shiny, soft hair is what we all want and as we age the opposite starts to happen. Why? You have to keep in mind that your hair reflects your overall health condition. It is crucial to fill your diet with proven hair growth nutrients and to improve your health from within. One of the first superfoods you should consume in order to prevent hair loss is definitely spinach. Because of its superior nutrient content, this is one of the best leafy green choices you can make when it comes to hair loss.

Hair loss and balding affect millions of men and women each year. One of the most common causes of hair loss, in both men and women, is malnutrition. The physical symptoms of hair loss can be traumatic, however the psychological impact is more severe. By increasing an intake of protein and iron, two of the most essential hair nutrients, and combining them with other essential nutrients hair loss can be reduced.

By simply changing a diet and increasing intake of Vitamins A, B, E, and K in addition to minerals selenium, phosphorus, magnesium, zinc, and niacin; anyone can have healthy hair. From promoting new growth to maintaining shine and body, these recipes are a guide for a new healthy lifestyle.

These meal and juice recipes will increase the nutrients necessary to help you strengthen your hair and make it vibrant again. Make these recipes part of your life and enjoy them every day!

77 HAIR LOSS PREVENTING MEAL AND JUICE RECIPES: USING HAIR GROWING VITAMINS AND MINERALS TO GIVE YOUR BODY THE TOOLS IT NEEDS

MEALS

1.   Grilled Chicken Skewers with Apricot

A year round summer dish, these skewers and be grilled or baked. When grilled, these skewers have a wonderful smoky sweet flavor and excess Vitamin A!

Ingredients:

- 2 boneless skinless chicken breast, cubed
- 1 red onion, cut into 1 inch cubes
- 1 red pepper, cut into 1 inch cubes
- 1 yellow pepper cut into 1 inch cubes
- 4 apricots, cut into quarters, pits removed
- 1 tablespoon olive oil
- 1 tablespoon honey
- 1/4 cayenne pepper

- 2 cups brown rice, cooked & hot

How to prepare:

Preheat grilled medium low.

Place one piece of chicken on skewer followed by onion, red pepper, yellow pepper and apricot. Repeat on skewer until no room remains. Repeat on remaining skewers until no ingredients remain.

Lightly brush skewers with olive oil. Place on grill. Cook for about 10 minutes, turning frequently until chicken is cooked through and vegetables are tender.

In small bowl, mix honey and cayenne. Brush on to skewers after they are cooked while they are hot. Serve skewers over brown rice.

Total calories: 645

Vitamins: Vitamin A 215 µg, Vitamin B6 1.7mg, Vitamin C 285mg

Minerals: Magnesium 163mg, Phosphorus 607mg, Selenium 65µg, Zinc 3mg, Niacin 28mg

Sugars: 12g

2.   Chicky Fried Rice

Instead of take out, try making this easy chicken fried rice from the comfort of your own kitchen! By adding more vegetables to the dish, extra nutrients are also added. This dish is also high in protein, each strand of hair is made of a protein complex. Making protein the base of all hair needs.

Ingredients:

- 2 eggs
- 2 tablespoon sesame oil
- 1 teaspoon fresh ginger, minced
- 2 cloves garlic, minced
- 1/4 teaspoon red pepper
- 1 small yellow onion, diced
- 4 boneless skinless chicken breast, diced
- 1/4 cup shredded carrot
- 1/4 cup sweet peas
- 2 tablespoon Hoisin sauce
- 4 cups brown rice, cooked
- 2 green onion, chopped
- 2 tablespoons fresh cilantro, chopped

How to prepare:

Lightly scramble eggs, set aside.

In large skillet, heat sesame oil on medium high heat. Add ginger, garlic, and red pepper and onion. Cook until fragrant and onion begins to soften. Add chicken, carrot and peas. Cook until no pink remains in the chicken. Add Hoisin sauce and brown rice, cook to heat through.

Once hot, add cooked scrambled eggs. Spoon into serving bowls and top with green onion and cilantro.

Total calories: 681

Vitamins: Vitamin B6 0.6mg

Minerals: Phosphorus 305mg, Selenium 47µg, Zinc 3mg, Niacin 8mg

Sugars: 2g

3.   Broccolini Pasta with Parmesan

If you like broccoli, you'll love broccolini! A hybrid of broccoli and kale, broccolini contains the nutrients of each vegetable. Giving it a healthy dose of Vitamins C and K – essential for proper hair growth.

Ingredients:

- 1 tablespoon olive oil
- 2 cups broccollini, chopped
- 2 clove garlic, minced
- 1/2 pound whole wheat linguini, cooked
- 2 tablespoons basil pesto
- 1/2 cup shredded parmesan

How to prepare:

In skillet, heat olive oil on medium heat. Add broccollini and garlic. Cook until broccollini is bright green and just beginning to soften. Add linguini and cook until hot. Stir in pesto and 3/4 of the parmesan. Spoon into bowls and top with remaining parmesan. Serve.

Total calories: 332

Vitamins: Vitamin C 40mg, Vitamin K 56 µg

Minerals: Phosphorus 266mg, Selenium 45µg

Sugars: 2g

4.   Orange Glazed Meatballs

Instead of regular every day meatballs – try making them with an easy twist! Orange gives this recipes a healthy dose of Vitamin C. Not only promoting healthy hair and skin, but giving these meatballs a zesty sweet finish.

Ingredients:

- 1 tablespoon olive oil
- 2 cups broccoli florets
- 1 pound extra lean ground beef
- 2 clove garlic
- 2 tablespoons Hoisin sauce, divided
- 2 tablespoons orange juice
- 2 teaspoons orange zest
- 1 tablespoon apple cider vinegar

How to prepare:

Preheat the oven to 400 degrees.

Place the broccoli baking sheet, drizzle with olive oil. Place in oven and cook or about 15 minutes, until tops just begin to brown.

Combine the ground beef, garlic, and half the hoisin sauce. Form into golf-ball-sized meatballs. In a large pan over medium high heat, add the meatballs Cook, rotating to brown all sides, for 5-7 minutes, or until cooked to desired doneness. Remove from the pan and set aside.

 Wipe out any burned bits from the pan. Returning it to medium-high heat, add the vinegar, orange juice, orange zest, and honey. Bring to a boil, then reduce to a simmer. Add broccoli and meatballs to the pan. Reduce until the sauce is thick and syrupy. Gently toss to coat everything in the glaze – sever over brown rice if desired.

Total calories: 477

Vitamins: Vitamin B6, 0.8mg, Vitamin B12 4.5 µg, Vitamin C 114mg, Vitamin K 95 µg

Minerals: Phosphorus 409mg, Selenium 35 µg, Zinc 10mg, Riboflavin 0.4mg, Niacin 10mg

Sugars: 13g

5.   Grilled Fish Tacos with Mango and Avocado

A taste of summer by the sea in each bite! Light and refreshing, these tacos are stuffed with Vitamin B and C giving you energy and healthy hair.

Ingredients:

- 1 tablespoon chili powder
- 2 teaspoons ground cumin
- 1 tablespoon paprika
- 1 teaspoon garlic powder
- 8 ounces Halibut
- 1 tablespoon olive oil
- 1/4 cup red cabbage, shredded
- 1 small onion, sliced
- 1 avocado, sliced
- 1/4 cup mango, diced
- 2 tablespoons fresh cilantro, chopped
- 1 tablespoon lime juice
- 4 small whole wheat tortillas

How to prepare:

In small bowl combine chili powder, cumin, paprika, and garlic powder. Lightly brush halibut with olive oil and coat well in spice mixture. In skillet on high heat, sear halibut until flaky. Remove from skillet and lightly break into smaller pieces.

Divide fish amongst tortillas. Top with remaining ingredients and drizzle of lime juice. Serve.

Total calories: 576

Vitamins: Vitamin B6 0.9mg, Vitamin B12 1.9 µg, Vitamin C 30mg, Vitamin E 7mg, Vitamin K 37 µg

Minerals: Magnesium 151mg, Phosphorus 586mg, Selenium 73 µg Thiamin 0.7mg, Niacin 9mg

Sugars: 8g

6.   Garlic Shrimp and Pasta with Vegetables

It's amazing how many nutrients are pack into a tiny shrimp. Paired with vegetables and whole wheat pasta, this easy dish is well rounded in filling, giving you all your body needs.

Ingredients:

- 1 tablespoon olive oil
- 12 ounces raw shrimp
- 3 cloves garlic, minced
- 1/4 cup onion, sliced
- 1/2 cup red bell pepper, sliced
- 1/2 cup zucchini, sliced
- 1/2 cup kale, chopped
- 1/4 cup skim milk
- 1/2 pound whole wheat penne pasta, cooked
- 1/2 cup shredded parmesan cheese

How to prepare:

In large skillet, heat oil on medium heat. Add shrimp, garlic, onion, bell pepper, and zucchini. Cook until shrimp are firm and pink. Add kale and cook until wilted.

Add milk and pasta to shrimp mix. Bring to a boil. Simmer and add parmesan cheese, stir until thickened. Spoon into bowls and serve.

Total calories: 697

Vitamins: Vitamin B6 0.7mg, Vitamin B12 2.3 µg, Vitamin C 49mg, Vitamin K 128 µg

Minerals: Magnesium 165mg, Phosphorus 808mg, Selenium 135 µg, Zinc 5mg

Sugars: 5

7.   Mediterranean Chicken Wrap

A great wrap for lunch or dinner, this light healthy option is stuffed with flavor and nutrients. In this dish, couscous makes this wrap filling while providing essential protein without the extra carbs.

Ingredients:

- 1/3 cup couscous, cooked
- 1 cup fresh parsley, chopped
- 2 tablespoons fresh oregano, chopped
- 1 tablespoon fresh mint, chopped
- 1/4 cup lemon juice
- 1 tablespoon olive oil
- 2 clove garlic, minced
- 3 boneless skinless chicken breast, sliced
- 1 medium tomato, chopped
- 1 small red onion, chopped
- 1 cup cucumber, chopped
- 4 tablespoons plain Greek yogurt
- 4 large whole wheat tortillas

How to prepare:

Combine parsley, oregano, mint, lemon juice, oil, garlic, in a small bowl. Pour 1/4 of the mixture over the chicken.

Coat the chicken well and cook in medium skillet until no pink remains.

Combine remaining parsley mixture with couscous. Add tomato, onion, cucumber and yogurt. Spoon onto tortillas and top with cooked chicken. Fold in sides of wrap and roll to form a burrito. Cut in half and serve.

Total calories: 349

Vitamins: Vitamin B6 0.8mg, Vitamin K 81 µg

Minerals: Phosphorus 391 mg, Selenium 44 µg, Zinc 2mg, Niacin 16mg

Sugars: 4g

8. Chicken, Broccoli, and Mango Stir fry

Spice up chicken and broccoli with sweet mango. Mango gives this classic dish added depth and flavor. Mango is packed with antioxidants, which help maintain collagen in the hair.

Ingredients:

- 2 tablespoons coconut oil
- 2 boneless skinless chicken breast, sliced
- 2 clove garlic, minced
- 1 tablespoon fresh ginger root, minced
- 1 small red onion, sliced
- 1 cup mango, sliced
- 2 cups broccoli, cut into small florets;
- 1/2 cup red bell pepper, chopped
- 3 tablespoons Hoisin sauce
- 1/4 teaspoon crush red pepper
- 1/4 cup cashews, chopped
- 3 green onion, chopped
- 1 tablespoon fresh cilantro, chopped

How to prepare:

Heat the coconut oil in a wok or skillet over medium-high heat.

Cook the chicken until no longer pink, and remove from skillet.

Add the garlic, ginger, and onion to same skillet. Cook until fragrant, about 1 to 2 minutes. Add the broccoli, bell pepper, and mango. Cook until the vegetables are just soft and still slightly crunch

Return the chicken to pan. Add Hoisin and red pepper flakes. Stir well to combine. Spoon into bowls. Sprinkle with chopped cashews, green onion, and cilantro. Serve.

Total calories: 357

Vitamins: Vitamin B6 0.8mg, Vitamin C 56 µg, Vitamin K 181 µg

Minerals: Phosphorus 248mg, Selenium 27 µg, Folate 165 µg, Riboflavin 0.4mg

Sugars: 21g

9.   Beef and Bok Choy Chow Mein

Little known box choy, or Asian Cabbage, is a great addition to any Asian dish! The nutrients in bok choy are similar to kale or other cabbage – giving recipes added nutrients and crunch!

Ingredients:

- 1 tablespoon coconut oil
- 12 ounces sirloin steak cubed
- 1 cup red onion, sliced
- 2 clove garlic, minced
- 1/2 cup red bell pepper, sliced
- 2 cups bok choy, chopped
- 1 cup bean sprouts
- 1/4 cup rice wine vinegar
- 2 tablespoons Hoisin Sauce
- 8 ounces soba noodles, cooked

How to prepare:

In large skillet or walk, heat oil on medium high heat. Add beef and cook until cooked through. Add onion, garlic, and peppers until vegetables just begin to soften. Add bok choy and cook until it beings to wilt. Add bean sprouts, vinegar and Hoisin, stir in noodles and toss to coat in sauce and heat through. Serve.

Total calories: 341

Vitamins: Vitamin B6 0.9mg, Vitamin C 70mg, Vitamin K 42 μg

Minerals: Phosphorus 348mg, Selenium 60 μg, Zinc 3mg, Thiamin 0.7mg, Riboflavin 0.5mg, Niacin 13mg

Sugars: 6g

10.   Seared Black Pepper Salmon with Cucumber Slaw

Pairing salmon with crisp cucumber slaw creates a balance of creamy and cool. Salmon provides healthy fats and Vitamin B, keeping hair healthy and shiny.

Ingredients:

- 1 tablespoon olive oil
- 2 (6 ounce) salmon filets
- 1/2 teaspoon salt
- 1/2 teaspoon black peppercorns, crushed
- 1/4 teaspoon crushed red pepper
- 1 cucumber, sliced thin
- 1/2 cup red cabbage, shredded
- 1/4 cup yellow onion, sliced thin
- 2/3 cup plain Greek Yogurt
- 1 teaspoon dry dill
- 1 clove garlic, minced
- 1 tablespoon apple cider vinegar

How to prepare:

In skillet, heat olive oil. Coat salmon with salt, peppercorns, and red pepper. Sear in skillet on medium high heat until firm and cooked through.

In medium bowl, combine remaining ingredients. Mix well. Allow to rest for 5 minutes. Spoon onto serving plate with salmon. Serve.

Total calories: 313

Vitamins: Vitamin B6 1.1mg, Vitamin B12 8.5 µg, Vitamin D 19 µg

Minerals: Phosphorus 566mg, Selenium 55 µg, Niacin 14mg

Sugars: 6g

11.   Avocado Egg Salad

Avocados contain the right combination of healthy fats and vitamins to encourage and improve hair growth. Supporting healthy blood flow, avocados also help improve cholesterol.

Ingredients

- 1/2 ripe avocado, pitted and peeled
- 1 boiled egg, peeled and chopped
- 2 tablespoons plain Greek yogurt
- 1/4 teaspoon crushed red pepper
- 1 teaspoon fresh parsley, chopped
- 1/4 cup fresh spinach
- 2 slices multigrain bread (toasted, if desired)

How to Prepare

With a fork, smash together all ingredients just until combined Serve between two slices of multigrain bread, top with spinach. Serve.

Total calories: 372

Vitamins: Vitamin B6 0.5mg, Vitamin E 5mg, Vitamin K 176 µg, Selenium 23 µg, Riboflavin 0.5mg

Sugars: 3g

12.   Spinach Orange Salad

Combining citrus and spinach is a classic combination. Orange pairs with the earthiness of the spinach; not only creating a balance of flavor and a well-rounded dish rich in vitamins and minerals.

Ingredients:

- 1 tablespoon olive oil
- 2 clove garlic, minced
- 2 tablespoons orange juice
- 2 boneless skinless chicken breast
- 1/4 cup balsamic vinegar
- 1 tablespoon honey
- 4 cups spinach
- 2 medium oranges, peeled and segmented
- 1/4 cup toasted almonds

How to prepare:

In small bowl, whisk together olive oil, garlic, and orange juice. Pour over chicken and marinate for 20 minutes.

Heat skillet on medium heat. Add chicken and cook through until no pink remains in the center. Set aside to rest.

In small sauce pot, bring vinegar and honey to a boil. Reduce to simmer. Continue to simmer, stirring occasionally, until sauce beings to thicken. Remove from heat and cool.

Divide spinach and oranges between serving bowls. Top with chicken. Sprinkle with almonds and drizzle with balsamic honey sauce. Serve.

Total calories: 399

Vitamins: Vitamin A 303 µg, Vitamin B6 1.0mg, Vitamin B12 0.4 µg, Vitamin C 87mg, Vitamin E 7mg, Vitamin K 290 µg

Minerals: Magnesium 150mg, Phosphorus 422mg, Selenium 36 µg, Niacin 19mg

Sugars: 13g

13. Roast Chicken Breast with Apricot Mustard and Swiss Chard

Chicken goes with everything, and apricot mustard and Swiss chard are an amazing combination! The zest of the mustard, sweetness of the apricot, and earthiness of the chard provides and out of this world experience sure to fulfill every vitamin and mineral need.

Ingredients:

- 1/4 cup fresh rosemary, chopped
- 3 clove garlic, minced & divided
- 2 tablespoons olive oil, divided
- 2 boneless skinless chicken breasts
- 1/4 cup grainy brown mustard
- 1/3 cup apricot jam
- 2 cups Swiss chard, chopped
- 1/2 cup onion, sliced

How to prepare:

Preheat oven to 350 degrees.

In a small bowl, combine the rosemary, 2/3 of the garlic, salt, and half the olive oil. Mix well. Rub chicken breast with the mixture.

Place chicken on cookie sheet. Cook 30 to 35 minutes, until no pink remains.

In a small saucepan, combine the mustard and apricot jam and heat over medium heat, stirring frequently, until jam has melted and ingredients are well combined.

Meanwhile, heat remaining oil in skillet on medium heat. Add remaining garlic, onion, and Swiss chard. Cook until Swiss chard is wilted and onions are soft. Spoon onto serving plate. Top with chicken and apricot glaze.

Total calories: 409

Vitamins: Vitamin A 611 µg, Vitamin B6 1.2mg, Vitamin C 32mg, Vitamin K 476 µg

Minerals: Magnesium 184mg, Phosphorus 451mg, Selenium 47 µg, Niacin 24mg

Sugars: 24g

14.   Blackened Salmon with Balsamic Kale

While kale contains any vitamins, this leafy green can become boring. Adding balsamic vinegar gives this vegetable new life! Paired with salmon, this recipe is loaded with Niacin, which helps convert food into healthy vitamins.

Ingredients:

- 2 tablespoons paprika
- 1 tablespoon cayenne pepper
- 1 tablespoon onion powder
- 1/2 teaspoon black pepper
- 1/4 teaspoon dried thyme
- 1/4 teaspoon dried oregano
- 1/4 teaspoon dried basil
- 2 tablespoons olive oil, divided
- 2 (6 ounces) salmon filets
- 3 cups kale, chopped
- 1 clove garlic, minced
- 1 tablespoon water
- 1 tablespoon balsamic vinegar

How to prepare:

Combine paprika, cayenne, onion powder, pepper, thyme, oregano, and basil in small bowl.

Brush salmon filets with half the olive oil. Coat salmon well with spice mix. Sear in skillet on medium heat, or grill on low heat, until fish is firm and flakey.

Heat remaining oil in skillet. Add kale, garlic, and water. Cook just until kale begins to wilt and stir in vinegar. Continue until liquid has evaporated. Spoon onto serving plate and top with salmon. Serve.

Total calories: 414

Vitamins: Vitamin A 602 µg, Vitamin B6 1.3mg, Vitamin B12 8.2 µg, Vitamin C 121mg, Vitamin D 19 µg, Vitamin K 729

Minerals: Phosphorus 552mg, Selenium 54 µg, Niacin 15mg

Sugars: 2g

15.   Lentil & Sweet Potato Calzone

Lentils are rich in many vitamins and minerals, too many to list! This key ingredient play a role in every aspect of hair growth – from the follicle to keeping hair strong and shiny.

Ingredients:

- 1 pizza crust, raw dough (preferably homemade)
- 3 small sweet potatoes,
- 2 tablespoons olive oil, divided
- 1 medium yellow onion, sliced
- 2 cloves garlic, minced
- 1 teaspoon ground cumin
- 1/2 teaspoon ground cinnamon
- 1/2 teaspoon ground allspice
- 1/2 cup French green lentils, rinsed
- 1 cup water
- 1 cup kale, chopped

How to prepare:

Preheat the oven to 400°F.

Prick the sweet potatoes in several places with a fork and place on a baking sheet. Bake 45 minutes to an hour, or until very soft to the touch. Allow to cool – once cool to the touch scoop out potato, mash and reserve. Throw out skins

Heat 1 tablespoon of oil in skillet over medium heat add onion and garlic. Cook until onion is translucent. Add the cumin, cinnamon, and allspice and cook, stirring, until fragrant. Add the lentils and water. Bring to a boil and simmer uncovered for 10 minutes. Add kale to lentil mix and continue to cook until lentils are soft but not mushy. If needed, add more water.

Increase the oven heat to 450°F.

On a well-floured cutting board, roll a piece of the dough into an 8- or 9-inch oval. Spread about 1/4 cup mashed sweet potato over bottom half the dough, leaving room at the edges to seal the pocket closed. Cover with about 1/3 cup of the lentils and kale. Fold top half of the dough over, and pinch and fold edges to seal securely.

Place on cookie sheet sprayed with nonstick spray. Brush top with olive oil and cut 2 or 3 small slits to let steam escape as it bakes. Repeat with remaining dough and filling.

Bake for 25 to 30 minutes, or until browned. Allow to rest for at least 5 minutes. Serve.

Total calories: 686

Vitamins: Vitamin A 1158 µg, Vitamin B6 0.7mg, Vitamin C 51mg, Vitamin K 256 µg

Minerals: Phosphorus 584mg, Selenium 24 µg, Folate 396 µg, Thiamin 0.8mg

Sugars: 12g

16.   Curried Egg Salad with Arugula on Rye

Tired of everyday egg salad? Adding curry gives boring egg salad a kick of spice! Adding arugula not only gives this sandwich a crisp crunch, but is full of Vitamin K! Pack this sandwich for lunch or eat for a quick dinner!

Ingredients:

- 4 hardboiled eggs, chopped
- 2 tablespoons celery, minced
- 2 tablespoon red onion, minced
- 1/2 teaspoon curry powder
- 3 tablespoons mayonnaise
- 2 tablespoons plain Greek yogurt
- 1/4 teaspoon Tabasco sauce
- 1 teaspoon Dijon mustard
- 4 slices rye bread, toasted
- 1/2 cup arugula

How to prepare:

Combine all ingredients with the exception of rye bread and arugula.

Divide the egg mix between two slices of rye. Top the egg mix with arugula and finish with second piece of rye bread. Cut in half and serve.

Total calories: 371

Vitamins: Vitamin A 184 µgm Vitamin B12 1.2 µg, Vitamin K 54 µg

Minerals: Phosphorus 292mg, Selenium 48 µg, Riboflavin 0.8mg

Sugars: 6g

17.   Bok Choy Egg Drop Soup

Adding bok choy to traditional egg drop soup extra vitamins in addition to the protein the soup already contains! Egg provide more than the minimum amount of daily protein, which is essential to proper hair growth.

Ingredients:

- 3 carrots, peeled and sliced
- 1 stalk celery, diced
- 1 small yellow onion, diced
- 1 clove garlic, minced
- 1 tablespoon fresh ginger, minced
- Pinch of Kosher or sea salt, more or less to taste
- 1/2 teaspoon black pepper
- 1 tablespoon chili powder
- 1/4 teaspoon cayenne pepper
- 1/4 teaspoon red pepper flakes (more if desired)
- 1 teaspoon paprika
- 4 cups chicken bone broth
- 2 tablespoons hoisin sauce
- 4 cups bok choy, chopped, loosely packed
- 4 egg whites
- 2 green onion, chopped
- 2 tablespoons fresh cilantro, chopped

How to prepare:

Add all ingredients, except bok choy, egg whites, green onion, and cilantro, to the slow cooker. Cover and cook on low 6 to 8 hours, or until the vegetables are tender. Add bok choy, stir and continue cooking just until wilted, approximately 5 minutes.

In a small bowl, whisk egg whites until frothy. Make sure the soup is hot and slowly stir while drizzling egg whites into the soup. Once all egg whites are incorporated, cook for an additional two minutes. Ladle into bowls, top with green onion and cilantro.

Total calories: 259

Vitamins: Vitamin A 837 µg, Vitamin B6 0.7mg, Vitamin C 69mg, Vitamin K 88 µg

Minerals: Phosphorus 225mg, Selenium 25 µg, Riboflavin 0.9mg, Niacin 9mg

Sugars: 14g

18. Root Vegetable and Lentil Soup with Poached Egg

A great fall soup, root vegetables are earthy and perfect for a cool day. Lentils make this a well-rounded dish while egg gives this soup a boost of protein.

Ingredients:

- 2 tablespoons olive oil
- 1 large onion, chopped
- 5 cloves garlic, minced
- 1 teaspoon ground cumin
- 1/2 teaspoon ground turmeric
- 6 slices turkey bacon, sliced
- 1 tablespoon fresh ginger, minced
- 1/2 teaspoon crushed red pepper
- 2 bay leaves
- 2 cups dried green lentils, rinsed
- 5 cups chicken bone broth (or vegetable broth)
- 1 (28-ounce) can crushed tomatoes
- 1 cup sweet potato, peeled and cubed
- 1 cup red beets, peeled and cubed
- 1 cup turnips, peeled and cubed
- 1 cup carrot, peeled and cubed
- 1 cup Idaho potatoes, peeled and cubed
- 4 raw eggs

- 3 cups water
- 2 tablespoons apple cider vinegar

How to prepare:

In an extra-large soup pot, heat the olive oil over medium heat and cook the onion until softened. Add the garlic, cumin and turmeric, mix well. Add the bacon. And cook until bacon browns, but is not crispy. Add the ginger, red pepper flakes, bay leaves, and lentils. Pour over enough stock to cover all ingredients. Bring to a boil cover and simmer for 15 minutes. Add remaining ingredients with the exception of eggs, water, and vinegar. Add more bone broth when needed, soup should be thick, but have some broth consistency. Continue to cook about 20 to 30 minutes until lentils and vegetables are tender but not falling apart. Remove bay leaves when cooked.

In small sauce pot, heat water and vinegar. Bring to a boil and reduce to a simmer. Swirl the water mix and while water is moving crack eggs into hot water one at a time. Remove from heat and allow to sit in hot wat for 5 to 8 minutes, depending on yolk preference. The longer in the water the harder the yolk.

Ladle soup into bowls. Using a slotted spoon, remove eggs – one at a time – and serve on top of soup.

Total calories: 333

Vitamins: Vitamin A 433 µg, Vitamin B6 0.6mg, Vitamin C 38mg

Minerals: Phosphorus 437mg, Selenium 20 µg, Zinc 3mg, Folate 304 µg

Sugars: 8g

19. Mediterranean Meatballs with Tzatziki and Couscous

A little known secret of the Mediterranean, meatballs with tangy yogurt sauce is a delicious end to any day! A quick and easy dinner entrée, this recipe is bursting with flavor.

Ingredients:

- 8 ounces ground lamb
- 8 ounces extra lean ground beef
- 6 cloves garlic, minced & divided
- 1 tablespoon dry oregano
- 2 tablespoon olive oil, divided
- 1/4 cup cucumber, shredded and drained of liquid
- 1 cup plain Greek yogurt
- 1 teaspoon dry dill
- 2 cups couscous, cooked and heated
- 1 lemon, cut into wedges

How to prepare:

Combine lamb, beef, half the garlic, and oregano. Form into balls. Heat half the olive oil in skillet on medium heat. Cook meatballs on all sides until no pink remains in center. Set aside.

Combine remaining garlic and oil with remaining ingredients with the exception of couscous and lemon.

Serve meatballs on top of couscous. Drizzle with yogurt sauce and serve with a lemon wedge.

Total calories: 349

Vitamins: Vitamin B12 3.2 µg

Minerals: Selenium 47 µg, Zinc 7mg, Niacin 8mg

Sugars: 3g

20.   Lentil & Sweet Potato Shepherd's Pie

A traditional Irish dish, this twist on Shepherd's pie is sure to leave you wanting more! This casserole and easy be made into individual servings and frozen for a later day.

Ingredients:

- 3 medium sweet potatoes, scrubbed
- 8 ounces extra lean ground beef
- 1 cup brown or green lentils, rinsed
- 1 tablespoon olive oil
- 1 pound cremini mushrooms, divided
- 1 medium yellow onion, chopped
- 1 large carrot, chopped
- 1 celery stalk, chopped
- 1 garlic clove, minced
- 3/4 cup low-sodium vegetable stock
- 1 tablespoon tomato paste
- 1 tablespoon Hoisin sauce
- 1 teaspoon smoked paprika
- 1/4 cup chopped fresh parsley

How to prepare:

Preheat the oven to 400 degrees. Prick each sweet potato several times with a fork and place on a baking sheet. Roast for 45 minutes to 1 hour, or until very soft to the touch. Set aside to cool. Once cool to the touch scoop out potato. Mash and reserve. Throw out peels. Reduce oven to 350 degrees.

In a medium pot, combine the lentils, bay leaf, and salt with 5 cups of water. Bring to a boil and lower heat. Simmer uncovered for 15-20 minutes, or until lentils are soft but not mushy, stirring occasionally. Discard bay leaf and drain mixture into a colander or sieve.

While the lentils are cooking, cook ground beef in skillet on medium heat. Once cooked completely and no pink remains add mushrooms and cook until browned and soft. Add onion, carrot, celery, and garlic and cook, stirring occasionally, until onions are soft and translucent. Lower heat to medium and add the lentil mix vegetable stock, tomato paste, Hoisin sauce, paprika, and parsley. Simmer mixture for 5 minutes.

Evenly spread the lentil mixture into a 9-x13-inch baking dish. Sprayed with nonstick spray. Spoon the sweet potato mixture on top and smooth with a spatula. Bake for 30 minutes, or until the filling is bubbling at the edges. Allow to rest for 5 minutes, serve.

Total calories: 406

Vitamins: Vitamin A 819 µg, Vitamin B6 0.8mg, Vitamin B12 2.3 µg µg

Minerals: Iron 7mg, Phosphorus 474mg, Selenium 22 µg, Zinc 7mg, Folate 267 µg, Niacin 7mg

Sugars: 8g

21. Slow Cooker Roasted Chicken with Root Vegetables

A blast from the past, this slow cooker chicken is sure to remind anyone of a home cooked Sunday meal. By preparing this meal in a slow cooker, it's great for a busy lifestyle and ensuring the proper amount of vitamins and minerals.

Ingredients:

- 1 whole chicken
- 1 tablespoon olive oil
- 1 tablespoon fresh sage, minced
- 1 tablespoon fresh rosemary, minced
- 2 clove garlic, minced
- 1 tablespoon fresh thyme, minced
- 1 sweet potato, peeled and cubed
- 1 carrot, peeled and cubed
- 1 turnip, peeled and cubed
- 4 red potatoes, quartered
- 1 small red onion, peeled and cubed
- 2 cups chicken bone broth

How to prepare:

Place chicken in slow cooker. Rub with olive oil, sage, rosemary, thyme and garlic. Arrange vegetables around chicken and pour broth over vegetables. Cook on low for 8 hours or high for 4 hours until vegetables are tender and no pink remains in chicken. Serve.

Total calories: 333

Vitamins: Vitamin A 371 µg, Vitamin B6 1.3mg, Vitamin B12 0.2 µg, Vitamin C 28mg

Minerals: Phosphorus 359mg, Selenium 30 µg, Zinc 2mg, Niacin 11mg

Sugars: 6g

22. Lemon Herb Salmon with Tomato Orzo

A fresh summer favorite, lemon provides a punch of Vitamin C a cuts the fatty texture of the salmon – which is packed with Vitamin B and Omega-3s. Omega-3s help give hair a healthy shine!

Ingredients:

- 2 tablespoons lemon juice
- 1 tablespoon Dijon mustard
- 2 cloves garlic, minced & divided
- 1/2 teaspoon dried dill
- 1/2 teaspoon dried oregano
- 1/4 teaspoon dried thyme
- 1/4 teaspoon dried rosemary
- 2 (6 ounce) salmon fillets
- 1 tablespoon olive oil
- 1/2 cup yellow onion, diced
- 2 cups water
- 1 (14 ounce) can diced tomatoes
- 1 cup orzo, dried
- 2 tablespoons chopped fresh parsley leaves

How to prepare:

Preheat oven to 375 degrees.

Combine lemon juice, Dijon, half the garlic, dill, oregano, thyme, and rosemary. Coat salmon with mixture. Place on cookie sheet sprayed with nonstick spray and bake for 10 to 15 minutes until fish is firm and flaky.

Meanwhile, heat olive oil in medium sauce pan on medium high heat. Cook onion and garlic until fragrant. Add water and bring to a boil. Once boiling, add tomatoes and orzo. Simmer, stirring frequently, until orzo is tender and water is evaporated. About 10 minutes. Spoon on to plate. Top with cooked salmon and fresh parsley. Serve.

Total calories: 622

Vitamins: Vitamin A 286 µg, Vitamin B6 2.4mg, Vitamin B12 19.1 µg, Vitamin C 23mg, Vitamin D 44 µg, Vitamin E 5mg

Minerals: Magnesium 139mg, Phosphorus 1108mg, Selenium 127 µg, Thiamin 0.8mg, Riboflavin 0.5mg, Niacin 34mg

Sugars: 4g

23. Steamed Mussels with Linguine, Spinach and Tomato

Change up pasta night with steamed mussels! Spinach and tomato ensure this pasta dish contains vitamin C while mussels provide selenium helps to maintain hair growth and prevent fallout.

Ingredients:

- 1 tablespoon olive oil
- 2 clove garlic, minced
- 2 tablespoons rice wine vinegar
- 1/4 cup water
- 1 pound mussels, cleaned
- 1 (14 ounce) can diced tomatoes
- 2 tablespoon fresh basil, minced
- 2 cups spinach
- 1/2 pound whole wheat linguini pasta, cooked
- 1/4 cup shredded parmesan

How to prepare:

In medium skillet, heat oil on medium high heat. Add garlic and cook until fragrant. Add vinegar, water, and mussels. Stir and cover until all mussel shells have opened, about 3 to 4 minutes. Remove and discard any mussels that remained closed.

Once mussels are cooked and diced tomatoes. Bring to a simmer and add basil and spinach. Cook until spinach is wilted and add pasta. Cook until heated through. Spoon into serving dishes and sprinkle with shredded parmesan.

Total calories: 506

Vitamins: Vitamin A 241 µg, Vitamin B6 0.6mg, Vitamin B12 17 µg, Vitamin C 39mg, Vitamin K 164 µg

Minerals: Magnesium 149mg, Phosphorus 467mg, Selenium 97mg, Zinc 4mg, Thiamin 1.6mg, Riboflavin 0.4mg

Sugars: 8g

24. Macadamia Crusted Chicken with Roasted Broccollini

A great alternative to everyday fried chicken! Macadamia nuts provide texture, flavor, and protein! Protein gives you hair strength, body, and bounce – ensure luscious locks!

Ingredients:

- 1 cup macadamia nuts, crushed fine
- 2 tablespoons grated parmesan cheese
- 2 tablespoon olive oil, divided
- 2 clove garlic, minced
- 2 small skinless boneless chicken breast
- 3 cups broccollini florets
- 1 tablespoon fresh basil, chopped

How to prepare:

Heat oven to 400 degrees.

Combine macadamia nuts, parmesan, half the olive oil, and garlic. Place chicken breast on cookie sheet sprayed with nonstick spray, leaving room for broccollini and press nut topping on to the top and sides of the chicken. Bake for 10 minutes.

Remove pan, and evenly spread broccollini on reserved pan space with chicken. Drizzle remaining olive oil on broccollini. Return pan to oven and bake an additional 10 minutes, until no pink remains in chicken and broccollini is crisp. Plate and serve, sprinkle with fresh basil.

Total calories: 646

Vitamins: Vitamin B6 0.9mg, Vitamin C 79mg, Vitamin K 90 µg

Minerals: Phosphorus 379mg, Selenium 33 µg, Thiamin 0.6mg, Niacin 13mg

Sugars: 4g

25. Spinach Salad with Spiced Carrots, Sunflower, and Salmon

Spice up salad with spiced carrots! Adding a punch of flavor, carrots provide a crunch and completes a well-rounded dish full of extra nutrients for preventing hair loss.

Ingredients:

- 2 carrots, shaved into long strips
- 1 tablespoon fresh ginger, grated
- 1/4 teaspoon chili powder
- 1 clove garlic, minced
- 1/4 teaspoon ground clove
- 1 tablespoon lime juice
- 1 teaspoon lime zest
- 1 tablespoon olive oil
- 3 teaspoon honey, divided
- 2 tablespoons apple cider vinegar
- 1 tablespoon apple juice
- 4 cups spinach
- 1/4 cup sunflower seeds

How to prepare:

Mix the carrots, ginger, chili powder, garlic, clove, lime and oil. Toss well to coat all carrots. Allow to rest.

Combine honey, vinegar, and juice in blender. Whisk together well to form a dressing. Pour over spinach and toss to coat. Place dressed spinach in bowls, top with sunflower seeds and carrots, serve.

Total calories: 265

Vitamins: Vitamin A 791 µg, Vitamin E 6mg, Vitamin K 298 µg

Minerals: Folate 166 µg

Sugars: 12g

26.   Rye and Arugula Poach Egg Sandwich

Creamy, crunchy, and packed with vitamins and minerals! Rye is highly nutritious, giving hair a boost of magnesium – which prevents unnecessary hair loss.

Ingredients:

- 1/4 cup feta cheese
- 2 tablespoons grated parmesan cheese
- 1/4 teaspoon dried thyme
- 1 tablespoon lemon juice, divided
- 3 cups water
- 2 tablespoons apple cider vinegar
- 2 eggs
- 1 cup arugula
- 1/4 teaspoon cayenne pepper

How to prepare:

Crumble the feta and mix with the Parmesan, thyme and half the lemon juice.

Toss the arugula and bean sprouts with oil and remaining lemon juice.

Bring water and vinegar to boil in medium sauce pot. Reduce to a simmer and swirl water to create movement.

While water continues to move, crack eggs one at a time into the water. Remove from heat and let sit for 5 to 8 minutes depend on doneness of yolk preference.

One each slice of rye bread, evenly top with arugula and bean sprouts. Followed by feta mix. With a slotted spoon, remove egg from water and place on top of feta. Sprinkle with cayenne and serve.

Total calories: 212

Vitamins: Vitamin B12 0.9mg

Minerals: Phosphorus 232mg, Selenium 28 µg, Riboflavin 0.5mg

Sugars: 2g

27. Garlic Lamb Chops with Lemon Kale and Sweet Potato

Lamb is not just for special occasions! Lamb is an outstanding source of zinc, iron, and Vitamin B12 and should be eaten more often. With sweet potato, this entrée promotes hair cell growth.

Ingredients:

- 2 sweet potatoes, peeled and cubed
- 2 tablespoons olive oil, divided
- 1 tablespoon fresh rosemary, chopped
- 10 ounces rack of lamb, cut into "lollipops"
- 4 clove garlic, minced & divided
- 1 tablespoon fresh oregano
- 3 cups kale, chopped
- 1 tablespoon water
- 1 tablespoon lemon juice
- 1 lemon, cut into wedges

How to prepare:

Preheat oven to 425 degrees

On cookie sheet sprayed with nonstick spray, arrange cubed sweet potato evenly. Sprinkle with half the olive oil and lightly toss. Bake in oven 30 to 40 minutes turning every 10 minutes, until soft and beginning to brown.

Meanwhile, coat lamb in half the garlic and oregano. Heat half of the remaining oil in skillet. Sear lamb, about 2 minutes each side to desired doneness. Lamb should be served slightly pink in the middle. Remove from pan and allow to rest.

In same skillet, heat remaining oil. Add remaining garlic, kale, water, and lemon juice. Cook until kale is wilted stirring frequently.

Serve sweet potatoes alongside kale and lamb on top of kale. Squeeze additional lemon juice on all items with lemon wedge. Serve.

Total calories: 639

Vitamins: Vitamin A 1257 µg, Vitamin B6 0.6mg, Vitamin B12 2.0 µg, Vitamin C 84mg, Vitamin K 478 µg

Minerals: Phosphorus 281mg, Selenium 24mg, Zinc 5mg, Niacin 6mg

Sugars: 5g

28.   Blueberry BBQ Chicken and Grilled Asparagus

Mix up traditional BBQ with a burst of blueberry! Also known as a superfood, blueberries are loaded with antioxidants which ensure healthy hair follicles and protects blood vessels to the follicles to promote healthy growth.

Ingredients:

- 3 cups fresh or frozen blueberries
- 1/4 cup tomato paste
- 1/2 cup cider vinegar
- 1/2 cup apple sauce
- 1/4 cup molasses
- 1 teaspoon chili powder
- 1 teaspoon ground black pepper
- 2 (8 ounce) boneless skinless chicken breast
- 1 tablespoon olive oil
- 1 pound asparagus

How to prepare:

Combine all ingredients, with exception of chicken, oil, and asparagus, in medium sauce pot. Bring to a boil, stirring frequently. Reduce and simmer – continue to stir every so often to break up blue berries. Allow to simmer for 20 minutes. If sauce becomes too thick, add a little water to thin. Strain out blueberry skins using cheese clothing or a fine mesh strainer.

Preheat grill to medium low heat. Lightly brush chicken with sauce. Place on grill – cook for 5 minutes and brush with more sauce. Turn chicken and cook an additional 5 minutes. Continue process until chicken is cooked through and no pink remains. Coat with additional sauce for serving.

Lightly toss asparagus in oil. Place on grill and cook for about 2 minutes. Serve alongside chicken.

Total calories: 463

Vitamins: Vitamin B6 1.3mg, Vitamin B12 0.6 µg, Vitamin C 23mg, Vitamin K 83 µg

Minerals: Phosphorus 471mg, Selenium 51 µg, Riboflavin 0.5mg, Niacin 25mg

Sugars: 36g

29.   Roasted Red Pepper and Goat Cheese Salad

Red peppers contain a large amount of Vitamin C, however not always a fan favorite when served raw. Try roasting red peppers and pairing them with a bit of salty bacon and creamy cheese!

Ingredients:

- 1 large red bell pepper
- 1 tablespoon olive oil
- 3 tablespoons balsamic vinegar
- 1 tablespoon honey
- 3 cups arugula
- 4 strips turkey bacon, cooked and chopped
- 1/4 cup goat cheese, crumbled
- 1/4 cup pecans, crushed
- 8 ounces skinless boneless chicken breast, cooked and chopped

How to prepare:

Preheat broiler to high temperature, about 500 degrees.

Cut the red pepper in half, removing seeds and white ribs. Brush the outside with olive oil and place on cookie sheet oil side up. Broil for 5 minutes, or until the outside of the peppers are charred and black. Place in bowl and cover with plastic wrap to cool. Once cool, scrape of charred skin and sliced into strips.

Meanwhile, combine vinegar in honey in sauce pot. Bring to a boil, stirring frequently, and simmer for about 2 minutes until sauce begins to thicken.

Divide arugula between two serving dishes. Top with red peppers and remaining ingredients. Drizzle with vinegar honey dressing and serve.

Total calories: 408

Vitamins: Vitamin A 227 µg, Vitamin B6 0.9mg, Vitamin B12 0.4 µg, Vitamin C 108mg

Minerals: Phosphorus 439mg, Selenium 30 µg, Niacin 13mg

Sugars: 5g

30.   Seared Ahi Tuna with Avocado Corn Salsa

Break from the norm with Ahi Tuna! A great source of B Vitamins and Omega-3s, Ahi pairs well with this simple corn salsa; which makes this entrée a well-rounded source of vitamins and minerals.

Ingredients:

- 2 (6 ounce) Ahi Tuna filets
- 1 tablespoon olive oil
- 1 teaspoon ground cumin
- 1 cup corn, cooked
- 1 jalapeño, seeded and diced
- 1/4 cup red onion, diced
- 2 tablespoons fresh cilantro, diced
- 2 tablespoons lime juice
- 2 Tomatoes, diced
- 1 avocado, halved, pit removed, peeled and diced
- 1/4 teaspoon Kosher salt

How to prepare:

Brush tuna with olive oil and dust with cumin. Sear in skillet on high heat, until outside is lightly browned and inside is still slightly pink, but firm.

Combine remaining ingredients, mix well. Allow to rest before serving on top of tuna.

Total calories: 422

Vitamins: Vitamin B6 2.0mg, Vitamin B12 3.5 µg, Vitamin C 62mg, Vitamin K 28 µg

Minerals: Phosphorus 579mg, Selenium 155 µg, Niacin 34mg

Sugars: 7g

31.   Broiled Chicken Gyro Salad

Love Gyros? You'll love this salad! For lunch or dinner, this Mediterranean delight is sure to please. Not only filling, leafy greens provide a daily dose of Vitamin K to promote hair growth.

Ingredients:

- 2 (6 ounce) boneless skinless chicken breast
- 2 tablespoon olive oil, divided
- 4 clove Garlic minced, divided
- 1 tablespoon fresh oregano, chopped
- 2 whole wheat pita, cut into triangles
- 1 teaspoon smoked paprika
- 1/4 cup cucumber, shredded
- 1 cup plan Greek yogurt
- 1 teaspoon dry dill
- 1 tablespoon water
- 1/4 cup romaine lettuce, chopped
- 1/4 cup arugula
- 1/4 cup spinach
- 1 tomato, sliced
- 1 small red onion, sliced
- 1/4 cup feta cheese

How to prepare:

Pre heat oven to 450

Combine chicken, half the oil, half the garlic, paprika, and oregano. Toss to coat chicken well. Place on cookie sheet until very crispy and cooked through. Remove from oven once cooked and slice into strips.

Lightly brush pita triangles with remaining olive oil. Bake in oven until crispy. About 5 to 10 minutes.

Meanwhile, combine remaining oil and garlic with cucumber, yogurt, and dill. Add enough water to make a dressing consistency.

Combine romaine, arugula, and spinach. Drizzle a few tablespoons of dressing and toss to coat. Divide amongst serving dishes and top with chicken and remaining ingredients. Serve with a side of pita chips and additional dressing if desired.

Total calories: 463

Vitamins: Vitamin B6 1.1mg, Vitamin K 127 µg

Minerals: Phosphorus 465mg, Selenium 57 µg, Niacin 19mg

Sugars: 4g

32.   Crispy Parmesan Chicken with Spinach

A healthier take on traditional parmesan chicken, this recipe cuts the fat and adds nutrition! In this dish, and abundance of phosphorus prevents hair fallout to help maintain a healthy scalp.

Ingredients:

- 2 tablespoon olive oil, divided
- 2 tablespoons whole wheat panko bread crumbs
- 1/4 cup shredded parmesan cheese
- 4 clove garlic, minced & divided
- 2 boneless skinless chicken breast
- 1/4 cup onion, chopped
- 2 cups spinach
- 1/2 cup diced tomatoes

How to prepare:

Preheat oven to 400 degrees.

Combine half the olive oil, panko, parmesan, and half the garlic. Lay chicken on cookie sheet sprayed with nonstick spray. Press panko and parmesan mix onto chicken breast, coating well Bake for 20 to 25 minutes until outside is brown and crispy and chicken is cooked through.

Meanwhile, in skillet heat remaining olive oil. Cook onion and remaining garlic on medium heat until onions soften. Add spinach and cook until wilted. Add tomato and cook until heated through. Spoon onto serving plate and top with chicken. Serve.

Total calories: 417

Vitamins: Vitamin B6 1.1mg, Vitamin B12 0.8 µg, Vitamin K 82µg

Minerals: Phosphorus 483mg, Selenium 49 µg, Niacin 24mg

Sugars: 8g

33. Southwest Black Bean Cakes with Arugula and Avocado

A great Tex-Mex recipe, black bean cakes are sure to please anyone! Black beans are a great source of protein, and arugula and avocado round out this dish with a selection of essential vitamins.

Ingredients:

- 1 tablespoon olive oil
- 1 red onion, minced
- 1 jalapeño pepper, minced
- 1/2 cup corn
- 2 cup black beans, cooked
- 1 roma tomato, diced
- 1 teaspoon ground cumin
- 1 teaspoon cayenne pepper
- 1/4 cup whole wheat panko breadcrumbs
- 1 avocado, pit removed, peeled, and cubed
- 1 cup arugula
- 4 tablespoons plain Greek yogurt
- 1 tablespoon balsamic vinegar
- 1 tablespoon lime juice
- 1 tablespoon fresh cilantro, chopped

How to Prepare:

Heat half the olive oil in a large skillet over medium heat. Add the half the onion and half the jalapeño to the pan. Cook until softened. Add the corn, black beans, cumin, cayenne, and half the tomato to the pan. Cook until softened. Remove from heat and pour mixture into a large bowl. Mash until nearly smooth. Stir in ¾ of the panko. Place the remaining panko into a small bowl. Form the black bean mixture into 2-inch patties, pressing each side into the panko.

Heat a drizzle of olive oil over medium heat. Once hot, add the black bean cakes to the pan. Cook 2-3 minutes per side, until golden brown.

In a medium bowl, combine the avocado, remaining tomato, remaining onion, and remaining jalapeño. Stir in lime juice.

In a medium bowl, toss the arugula with balsamic vinegar. Serve the smoky black bean cakes on a bed of arugula. Top with the avocado salsa and a dollop of Greek yogurt and cilantro.

Total calories: 434

Vitamins: Vitamin K 33 μg

Minerals: Phosphorus 245mg Zinc 3mg, Thiamin 0.4mg

JUICES

1. Orange Celery Juice

Ingredients:

1 small orange, wedged

2 medium-sized celery stalk

1 small apple, cored

1 large strawberry, chopped

Preparation:

Peel the orange and divide into wedges. Set aside.

Wash the celery and cut into bite-sized pieces. Set aside.

Wash the apple and cut in half. Remove the core and cut into bite-sized pieces. Set aside.

Wash the strawberry and cut in half. Set aside.

Now, combine orange, celery, apple, and strawberry in a juicer and process until well juiced. Transfer to a serving glass and add some crushed ice.

Serve immediately.

Nutrition information per serving: Kcal: 116, Protein: 2.2g, Carbs: 34.6g, Fats: 0.6g

2.   Cauliflower Carrot Juice

Ingredients:

2 cauliflower flowerets, chopped

2 small carrots, chopped

1 cup of blackberries

1 cup of cucumber, sliced

1 cup of fresh kale, torn

Preparation:

Wash the cauliflower thoroughly and chop into small pieces. Set aside.

Wash and peel the carrots. Cut into thin slices and set aside.

Place the blackberries in a colander and rinse under cold running water. Slightly drain and set aside.

Wash the cucumber and cut into thin slices. Fill the measuring cup and reserve the rest for later.

Rinse the kale thoroughly and slightly drain. Torn with hands and set aside.

Now, combine cauliflower, carrots, blackberries, cucumber, and kale in a juicer and process until juiced.

Transfer to a serving glass and serve cold.

Nutrition information per serving: Kcal: 94, Protein: 6.4g, Carbs: 32.5g, Fats: 1.7g

3.   Orange Lemon Juice

Ingredients:

1 large orange, wedged

2 whole lemons, peeled

1 whole lime, peeled

1 small ginger slice, peeled

1 oz. of water

Preparation:

Peel the orange and divide into wedges. Cut each wedge in half and set aside.

Peel the lemons and lime. Cut each fruit lengthwise in half and set aside.

Peel the ginger slice and set aside.

Now, combine orange, lemons, lime, and ginger in a juicer and process until well juiced. Add some ice and water to the juicer and blend again.

Transfer to a serving glass and garnish with some lemon or lime slices before serving.

Enjoy!

Nutrition information per serving: Kcal: 102, Protein: 3.3g, Carbs: 36.5g, Fats: 0.6g

4.   Avocado Broccoli Juice

Ingredients:

1 cup of avocado, cubed

1 cup of broccoli, chopped

1 small zucchini, cubed

1 cup of pomegranate seeds

Preparation:

Peel the avocado cut lengthwise in half. Remove the pit and cut into small cubes. Fill the measuring cup and reserve the rest for later. Set aside.

Wash the broccoli and cut into small pieces. Set aside.

Wash and peel the zucchini. Cut into small cubes and set aside.

Cut the top of the pomegranate fruit using a sharp paring knife. Slice down to each of the white membranes inside of the fruit. Pop the seeds into a measuring cup and set aside.

Now, combine avocado, broccoli, zucchini, and pomegranate seeds in a juicer and process until juiced.

Transfer to a serving glass and add some ice before serving. Garnish with some fresh mint, if you like. However, it's optional.

Enjoy!

Nutrition information per serving: Kcal: 294, Protein: 8.5g, Carbs: 38.7g, Fats: 23.7g

5.   Mango Mint Juice

Ingredients:

1 cup of mango, cubed

1 cup of fresh mint, torn

1 large banana, sliced

1 whole grapefruit, wedged

1 oz. of coconut water

Preparation:

Peel the mango and cut into small cubes. Fill the measuring cup and reserve the rest for later.

Wash the mint thoroughly and torn with hands. Set aside.

Peel the banana and cut into thin slices. Set aside.

Peel the grapefruit and divide into wedges. Cut each wedge in half and set aside.

Now, combine mango, mint, banana, and grapefruit in a juicer and process until juiced. Transfer to a serving glass and stir in the coconut water. Add some ice and serve immediately.

Enjoy!

Nutrition information per serving: Kcal: 293, Protein: 5.6g, Carbs: 85.7g, Fats: 1.6g

6. Coriander Spinach Juice

Ingredients:

1 cup of fresh coriander, chopped

1 cup of fresh spinach, torn

1 cup of Romaine lettuce, shredded

1 whole cucumber, sliced

¼ tsp of salt

Preparation:

Combine coriander, spinach, and lettuce in a large colander. Wash thoroughly under cold running water and slightly drain. Roughly chop all and set aside.

Wash the cucumber and cut into thin slices. Set aside.

Now, combine coriander, spinach, lettuce, and cucumber in a juicer and process until well juiced.

Transfer to a serving glass and stir in the salt.

Serve immediately.

Nutrition information per serving: Kcal: 85, Protein: 10.3g, Carbs: 23.9g, Fats: 1.8g

7. Carrot Lime Juice

Ingredients:

2 medium-sized carrots, sliced

1 whole lime, peeled

1 cup of cucumber, sliced

1 medium-sized orange, wedged

1 tbsp. of honey

Preparation:

Wash and peel the carrots. Cut into thin slices and set aside.

Peel the lime and cut lengthwise in half. Set aside.

Wash the cucumber and cut into thin slices. Fill the measuring cup and reserve the rest for later.

Peel the orange and divide into wedges. Cut each wedge in half and set aside.

Now, combine carrots, lime, cucumber, and orange in a juicer and process until juiced. Transfer to a serving glass and stir in the honey.

Add some ice before serving.

Enjoy!

Nutrition information per serving: Kcal: 163, Protein: 2.9g, Carbs: 32.6g, Fats: 0.6g

8.   Beet Grapefruit Juice

Ingredients:

1 cup of beets, trimmed and sliced

1 whole grapefruit, peeled

1 cup of avocado, cubed

½ cup of green grapes

Preparation:

Wash the beets thoroughly and trim off the green parts, cut into thin slices and fill the measuring cup. Reserve the rest in the refrigerator.

Peel the grapefruit and divide into wedges. Cut each wedge in half and set aside.

Peel the avocado and cut lengthwise in half. Cut into small cubes and fill the measuring cup. Reserve the rest for later.

Wash the grapes and fill the measuring cup. Set aside.

Now, combine beets, grapefruit, avocado, and grapes in a juicer. Add few ice cubes and process until juiced.

Transfer to a serving glass and serve immediately.

Nutrition information per serving: Kcal: 350, Protein: 7.3g, Carbs: 56.1g, Fats: 22.6g

9. Tomato Parsley Juice

Ingredients:

5 cherry tomatoes, halved

1 cup of fresh parsley, finely chopped

1 cup of cucumber, sliced

1 large red bell pepper, chopped

1 whole lemon, peeled

1 tsp of fresh rosemary, finely chopped

Preparation:

Wash the cherry tomatoes and place in a bowl. Cut each tomato in half and make sure to reserve the tomato juice.

Wash the parsley thoroughly under cold running water and slightly drain. Roughly chop it and set aside.

Wash the cucumber and cut into thin slices. Fill the measuring cup and reserve the rest for later.

Wash the bell pepper and cut in half. Remove the seeds and chop into small pieces. Set aside.

Peel the lemon and cut lengthwise in half. Set aside.

Now, combine cherry tomatoes, parsley, cucumber, bell pepper, lemon, and rosemary in a juicer and process until well juiced. Transfer to a serving glass and refrigerate for 10 minutes before serving.

Nutrition information per serving: Kcal: 79, Protein: 5.1g, Carbs: 24.9g, Fats: 1.3g

10.   Mango Banana Juice

Ingredients:

1 cup of mango, chunked

1 medium-sized banana, sliced

1 small apple, cored

1 cup of fresh mint, torn

1 small ginger knob, peeled

1 tbsp. of liquid honey

Preparation:

Peel the mango and cut into small chunks. Fill the measuring cup and reserve the rest for later. Set aside.

Peel the banana and cut into thin slices. Set aside.

Wash the apple and cut in half. Remove the core and cut into bite-sized pieces. Set aside.

Place the mint in a large colander. Rinse well under cold running water and slightly drain. Torn with hands and set aside.

Peel the ginger knob and set aside.

Now, combine mango, banana, apple, mint, and ginger in a juicer and process until juiced. Transfer to a serving glass and stir in the honey.

Add few ice cubes and serve immediately.

Nutrition information per serving: Kcal: 325, Protein: 4.3g, Carbs: 76.1g, Fats: 1.6g

11.   Broccoli Cabbage Juice

Ingredients:

1 cup of broccoli, chopped

1 cup of purple cabbage, torn

1 whole beet, chopped

1 cup of Swiss chard, torn

1 cup of cucumber, sliced

¼ tsp of turmeric, ground

Preparation:

Wash the broccoli and trim off the outer layers. Chop it into small pieces and set aside.

Combine purple cabbage and Swiss chard in a large colander. Wash thoroughly under cold running water and slightly drain. Torn with hands and set aside.

Wash the beets and trim off the green parts. Cut into bite-sized pieces and set aside.

Wash the cucumber and cut into thin slices. Fill the measuring cup and reserve the rest for later. Set aside.

Now, combine broccoli, purple cabbage, beet, Swiss chard, and cucumber in a juicer and process until juiced.

Transfer to a serving glass and stir in the turmeric. Refrigerate for 15 minutes and serve.

Enjoy!

Nutrition information per serving: Kcal: 79, Protein: 6.2g, Carbs: 23.7g, Fats: 0.8g

12.   Artichoke Orange Juice

Ingredients:

1 medium-sized artichoke, chopped

1 small orange, peeled

1 whole lemon, peeled

1 whole lime, peeled

1 tbsp. of liquid honey

1 oz. of water

Preparation:

Trim off the outer layers of the artichoke using a sharp paring knife. Cut into bite-sized pieces and set aside.

Peel the orange and divide into wedges. Cut each wedge in half and set aside.

Peel the lemon and lime. Cut each fruit lengthwise in half and set aside.

Now, combine artichoke, orange, lemon, and lime in a juicer. Process until well juiced. Transfer to a serving glass and stir in the honey and water.

Refrigerate for 10 minutes before serving.

Nutrition information per serving: Kcal: 149, Protein: 5.9g, Carbs: 33.8g, Fats: 0.5g

13. Honeydew Melon Juice

Ingredients:

1 medium-sized slice of honeydew melon

1 medium-sized carrot, sliced

1 medium-sized peach, chopped

1 small green apple, cored

Preparation:

Cut melon lengthwise in half. Scoop out the seeds and then wash the melon. Cut one wedge and peel it. Cut into bite-sized pieces and set aside.

Wash and peel the carrot. Cut into thin slices and set aside.

Wash the peach and cut in half. Remove the pit and cut small pieces. Set aside.

Wash the apple and cut in half. Remove the core and cut into bite-sized pieces. Set aside.

Now, combine melon, carrot, peach, and apple in a juicer and process until juiced. Transfer to a serving glass and refrigerate for 10 minutes before serving.

Nutrition information per serving: Kcal: 176, Protein: 3.2g, Carbs: 51.1g, Fats: 1g

14.   Blueberry Lemon Juice

Ingredients:

1 cup of blueberries

1 whole lemon, peeled

1 large banana, sliced

1 large pear, chopped

2 oz of coconut water

Preparation:

Place the blueberries in a colander and rinse under cold water. Slightly drain and set aside.

Peel the lemon and cut lengthwise in half. Set aside.

Peel the banana and cut into thin slices. Set aside.

Wash the pear and cut in half. Remove the core and cut into bite-sized pieces. Set aside.

Now, combine blueberries, lemon, banana, and pear in a juicer and process until juiced. Transfer to a serving glass and stir in the coconut water. Add some ice and serve immediately.

Enjoy!

Nutrition information per serving: Kcal: 291, Protein: 4.1g, Carbs: 92.3g, Fats: 1.4g

15.   Cherry Cantaloupe Juice

Ingredients:

1 cup of cherries, pitted

1 small cantaloupe wedge

1 whole lemon, peeled

1 cup of pineapple chunks

Preparation:

Wash the cherries and remove the green stems, if any. Cut each cherry in half and fill the measuring cup. Set aside.

Cut the cantaloupe in half. Scrape out the seeds and cut one thin slice. Wrap the rest in a plastic foil and refrigerate for later.

Peel the lemon and cut lengthwise in half. Set aside.

Using a sharp paring knife, cut the top of the pineapple. Gently remove all hard skin and slice it into thin slices. Fill the measuring cup and reserve the rest for later.

Now, combine cherries, cantaloupe, lemon, and pineapple in a juicer. Process until well juiced. Transfer to a serving glass and refrigerate for 10 minutes before serving. Enjoy!

Nutrition information per serving: Kcal: 176, Protein: 3.4g, Carbs: 53.6g, Fats: 0.7g

16.   Pepper Greens Juice

Ingredients:

1 large red bell pepper, chopped

1 cup of collard greens, chopped

1 cup of fennel, chopped

1 large radish, chopped

1 whole lemon, peeled

1 small ginger knob, peeled

1 oz of water

Preparation:

Wash the bell pepper and cut in half. Remove the seeds and chop into small pieces. Set aside.

Wash the collard greens and chop into small pieces. Set aside.

Trim off the outer wilted layers of the fennel. Roughly chop it and fill the measuring cup. Reserve the rest for later.

Wash the radish and trim off the green ends. Slightly peel it and chop into small pieces. Set aside.

Peel the lemon and cut lengthwise in half. Set aside.

Peel the ginger knob and roughly chop it. Set aside.

Now, combine bell pepper, collard greens, fennel, radish, lemon, and ginger in a juicer. Process until juiced.

Transfer to a serving glass and stir in the water. Refrigerate for 10 minutes before serving.

Nutrition information per serving: Kcal: 76, Protein: 4.6g, Carbs: 24.9g, Fats: 1.1g

17.   Cauliflower Kale Juice

Ingredients:

1 cup of cauliflower, chopped

1 cup of fresh kale, chopped

1 whole lime, peeled

1 cup of cucumber, sliced

¼ tsp of salt

Preparation:

Trim off the outer layer of the cauliflower. Cut into bite-sized pieces and wash it. Fill the measuring cup and sprinkle with some salt. Set aside.

Wash the kale thoroughly under cold running water and slightly drain. Chop into small pieces and set aside.

Peel the lime and cut lengthwise in half. Set aside.

Wash the cucumber and cut into thin slices. Fill the measuring cup and reserve the rest for some other juice. Set aside.

Now, combine cauliflower, kale, lime, and cucumber in a juicer. Process until well juiced. Transfer to a serving glass and refrigerate before serving.

Enjoy!

Nutrition information per serving: Kcal: 87, Protein: 11.4g, Carbs: 24.4g, Fats: 1.8g

18. Avocado Carrot Juice

Ingredients:

1 cup of avocado, chunked

1 large carrot, sliced

1 small red apple, cored

½ cup of green grapes

1 whole kiwi, peeled

¼ tsp of ginger, ground

Preparation:

Peel the avocado and cut in half. Remove the pit and cut into small chunks. Fill the measuring cup and reserve the rest for later.

Wash and peel the carrot. Cut into thin slices and set aside.

Wash the apple and cut in half. Remove the core and cut into bite-sized pieces. Set aside.

Peel the kiwi and cut lengthwise in half. Set aside.

Now, combine avocado, carrot, apple, grapes, and kiwi in a juicer and process until juiced. Transfer to a serving glass and stir in the ginger.

Add some crushed ice and serve immediately.

Nutrition information per serving: Kcal: 355, Protein: 5.1g, Carbs: 56.1g, Fats: 22.9g

19.   Grapefruit Cherry Juice

Ingredients:

1 whole grapefruit, peeled

1 cup of cherries, pitted

1 medium-sized banana, sliced

1 cup of fresh mint, torn

2 tbsp. of coconut water

Preparation:

Peel the grapefruit and divide into wedges. Cut each wedge in half and set aside.

Wash the cherries and remove the stems, if any. Cut each cherry in half and remove the pits. Fill the measuring cup and set aside.

Peel the banana and cut into thin slices. Set aside.

Wash the mint thoroughly under cold running water and slightly drain. Torn with hands and set aside.

Now, combine grapefruit, cherries, banana, and mint in a juicer and process until juiced. Transfer to a serving glass and stir in the coconut water.

Add some crushed ice and serve immediately.

Nutrition information per serving: Kcal: 274, Protein: 5.8g, Carbs: 81.5g, Fats: 1.3g

20.   Apple Kiwi Juice

Ingredients:

1 small apple, cored

1 whole kiwi, peeled

 1 small peach, pitted

½ cup of fresh spinach, torn

Preparation:

Wash the apple and cut in half. Remove the core and cut into bite-sized pieces. Set aside.

Peel the kiwi and cut lengthwise in half. Set aside.

Wash the peach and cut in half. Remove the pit and cut into bite-sized pieces. Set aside.

Rinse the spinach under cold running water and slightly drain. Torn with hands and set aside.

Now, combine apple, kiwi, peach, and spinach in a juicer and process until juiced. Transfer to a serving glass and add some ice.

Serve immediately.

Nutrition information per serving: Kcal: 165, Protein: 6.9g, Carbs: 47.6g, Fats: 1.5g

21.   Parsnip Beet Juice

Ingredients:

1 cup of parsnip, sliced

1 cup of beets, sliced

1 cup of sweet potatoes, chunked

1 cup of mustard greens, torn

1 cup of watercress, torn

Preparation:

Wash and peel the parsnips. Remove the green parts and cut into thin slices. Fill the measuring cup and reserve the rest for later.

Wash the beets and trim off the green ends. Slightly peel and cut into thin slices. Fill the measuring cup and set aside.

Peel the potato and cut into small chunks. Fill the measuring cup and reserve the rest for later.

Combine mustard greens and watercress in a colander. Wash thoroughly under cold running water and slightly drain. Torn with hands and set aside.

Now, combine parsnips, beets, sweet potatoes, mustard greens, and watercress in a juicer and process until juiced.

Transfer to a serving glass and add some salt if you like. However, it is optional.

Nutrition information per serving: Kcal: 226, Protein: 8.3g, Carbs: 66.7g, Fats: 0.9g

22.   Watermelon Blackberry Juice

Ingredients:

1 cup of watermelon, cubed

1 cup of blackberries

1 medium-sized orange, peeled

1 tbsp of liquid honey

¼ tsp of cinnamon, ground

Preparation:

Cut the watermelon in half. Cut one large wedge and wrap the rest in a plastic foil and refrigerate. Peel the slice and cut into small cubes. Remove the pits and fill the measuring cup. Set aside.

Wash the blackberries thoroughly under cold water and slightly drain. Set aside.

Peel the orange and divide into wedges. Cut each wedge in half and set aside.

Now, combine watermelon, blackberries, and orange in a juicer and process until juiced. Transfer to a serving glass and stir in the honey and cinnamon.

Refrigerate for 10 minutes before serving.

Enjoy!

Nutrition information per serving: Kcal: 186, Protein: 4.2g, Carbs: 40.7g, Fats: 1.1g

23.   Cranberry Raspberry Juice

Ingredients:

1 cup of cranberries

1 cup of raspberries

1 cup of fresh mint, torn

1 whole lemon, peeled

1 small apple, cored

Preparation:

Combine cranberries and raspberries in a large colander. Wash thoroughly under cold running water and slightly drain. Set aside.

Wash the mint and torn with hands. Set aside.

Peel the lemon and cut lengthwise in half. Set aside.

Wash the apple and cut in half. Remove the core and cut into bite-sized pieces.

Now, combine cranberries, raspberries, mint, lemon, and apple in a juicer and process until juiced. Transfer to a serving glass and add some ice before serving.

Enjoy!

Nutrition information per serving: Kcal: 143, Protein: 3.8g, Carbs: 53.5g, Fats: 1.5g

24. Strawberry Banana Juice

Ingredients:

1 cup of strawberries, chopped

1 medium-sized banana, sliced

1 whole grapefruit, wedged

1 small Granny Smith's apple, cored

1 tbsp of coconut water

Preparation:

Wash the strawberries and remove the stems. Cut into bite-sized pieces and fill the measuring cup. Reserve the rest for later.

Peel the banana and cut into thin slices. Set aside.

Peel the grapefruit and divide into wedges. Cut each wedge in half and set aside.

Wash the apple and cut lengthwise in half. Remove the core and cut into bite-sized pieces. Set aside.

Now, combine strawberries, banana, grapefruit, and apple in a juicer and process until well juiced. Transfer to a serving glass and stir in the coconut water.

Add few ice cubes and serve immediately.

Nutrition information per serving: Kcal: 268, Protein: 4.4g, Carbs: 79.6g, Fats: 1.2g

25.   Guava Mango Juice

Ingredients:

1 whole guava, peeled

1 medium-sized orange, peeled

1 large carrot, sliced

1 whole lemon, peeled

1 tbsp of liquid honey

Preparation:

Peel the guava with a sharp paring knife. Cut into small chunks and set aside.

Peel the orange and divide into wedges. Cut each wedge in half and set aside.

Wash and peel the carrot. Cut into thin slices and set aside.

Peel the lemon and cut lengthwise in half. Set aside.

Now, combine guava, orange, carrot, and lemon in a juicer and process until juiced. Transfer to a serving glass and stir in the honey. Add some ice and serve immediately.

Nutrition information per serving: Kcal: 168, Protein: 3.9g, Carbs: 35.6g, Fats: 1.1g

26.   Pineapple Cherry Juice

Ingredients:

1 cup of pineapple, chunked

1 cup of cherries, pitted

1 medium-sized carrot, sliced

¼ tsp of ginger, ground

1 tbsp of coconut water

Preparation:

Using a sharp paring knife, cut the top of the pineapple. Gently remove all hard skin and slice it into thin slices. Fill the measuring cup and reserve the rest for later.

Wash the cherries and cut each in half. Remove the pits and fill the measuring cup. Reserve the rest in the refrigerator.

Wash and peel the carrot. Cut into thin slices and set aside.

Now, combine pineapple, cherries, and carrot in a juicer and process until well juiced. Transfer to a serving glass and stir in the ginger and coconut water. Garnish with some fresh mint and serve immediately.

Nutrition information per serving: Kcal: 175, Protein: 3.1g, Carbs: 52.1g, Fats: 0.6g

27. Zucchini Asparagus Juice

Ingredients:

1 small zucchini, chopped

2 medium-sized asparagus spears

1 cup of celery, chopped

1 cup of fresh basil, torn

1 whole lime, peeled

Preparation:

Wash the zucchini and cut into bite-sized pieces. Set aside.

Wash the asparagus and trim off the woody ends. Cut into small pieces and set aside.

Wash the celery and remove the white parts. Cut the green parts into small pieces. Set aside.

Rinse the basil under cold running water using a colander. Slightly drain and torn with hands. Set aside.

Peel the lime and cut lengthwise in half. Set aside.

Now, combine zucchini, asparagus, celery, basil, and lime in a juicer and process until juiced. Transfer to a serving glass and add some ice before serving.

Enjoy!

Nutrition information per serving: Kcal: 43, Protein: 3.7g, Carbs: 12.3g, Fats: 0.7g

28.   Mango Pear Juice

Ingredients:

1 cup of mango, chunked

1 medium-sized pear, chopped

1 cup of pomegranate seeds

1 cup of Romaine lettuce, shredded

1 tbsp. of liquid honey

Preparation:

Peel the mango and cut into small chunks. Fill the measuring cup and reserve the rest in the refrigerator. Set aside.

Wash the pear and cut into small pieces. Set aside.

Cut the top of the pomegranate fruit using a sharp paring knife. Slice down to each of the white membranes inside of the fruit. Pop the seeds into a measuring cup and set aside.

Wash the lettuce thoroughly under cold running water and shred it. Fill the measuring cup and reserve the rest for later.

Now, combine mango, pear, pomegranate, and lettuce in a juicer and process until well juiced. Transfer to a serving glass and stir in the honey. Add some ice and serve immediately.

Nutrition information per serving: Kcal: 230, Protein: 4.1g, Carbs: 69.6g, Fats: 2.1g

29.   Plum Kiwi Juice

Ingredients:

2 large plums, pitted

1 whole kiwi, peeled

1 cup of cantaloupe, chunked

1 cup of red leaf lettuce, shredded

1 tbsp of liquid honey

Preparation:

Wash the plums and cut in half. Remove the pits and cut into bite-sized pieces. Set aside.

Peel the kiwi and cut lengthwise in half. Set aside.

Cut the cantaloupe in half. Scoop out the seeds and flesh. Cut two wedges and peel them. Chop into chunks and set aside. Reserve the rest of the cantaloupe in a refrigerator.

Wash the lettuce thoroughly and shred it. Fill the measuring cup and reserve the rest for later.

Now, combine plums, kiwi, cantaloupe, and lettuce in a juicer and process until juiced. Transfer to a serving glass and stir in the honey.

Add some ice and serve immediately.

Nutrition information per serving: Kcal: 136, Protein: 3.4g, Carbs: 38.6g, Fats: 1.1g

30.   Basil Tomato Juice

Ingredients:

1 cup of fresh basil, torn

5 cherry tomatoes, halved

1 cup of fresh parsley, torn

1 cup of fresh spinach, chopped

1 cup of mustard greens, torn

¼ tsp of salt

Preparation:

Combine basil, parsley, and mustard greens in a colander. Rinse well under cold running water and slightly drain. Torn with hands and set aside.

Wash the spinach leaves and chop into small pieces. Fill the measuring cup and reserve the rest for later. Set aside.

Wash the cherry tomatoes and remove the stems. Place in a small bowl and cut in half. Make sure to reserve the juice while cutting. Set aside.

Now, combine basil, parsley, mustard greens, spinach and tomatoes in a juicer and process until well juiced. Transfer to a serving glass and stir in the reserved tomato juice and salt.

Serve cold.

Nutrition information per serving: Kcal: 64, Protein: 10.9g, Carbs: 17.9g, Fats: 1.8g

31.   Orange Cantaloupe Juice

Ingredients:

1 large orange, peeled

1 medium-sized slice of cantaloupe

1 small ginger knob, peeled

1 cup of cucumber, sliced

1 tbsp of coconut water

Preparation:

Peel the orange and divide into wedges. Cut each wedge in half and set aside.

Cut the cantaloupe in half. Scoop out the seeds and cut the wedge. Peel it and cut into small pieces. Set aside.

Peel the ginger knob and cut in small pieces. Set aside.

Wash the cucumber and cut into thin slices. Fill the measuring cup and reserve the rest for later. Set aside.

Now, combine orange, cantaloupe, ginger, and cucumber in a juicer and process until juiced. Transfer to a serving glass and stir in the coconut water.

Refrigerate for 10 minutes before serving.

Nutrition information per serving: Kcal: 103, Protein: 2.7g, Carbs: 30.2g, Fats: 0.5g

32.   Pomegranate Watermelon Juice

Ingredients:

1 cup of pomegranate seeds

1 cup of watermelon, cubed

1 whole beet, sliced

1 cup of watercress, torn

Preparation:

Cut the top of the pomegranate fruit using a sharp paring knife. Slice down to each of the white membranes inside of the fruit. Pop the seeds into a measuring cup and set aside.

Cut the watermelon lengthwise in half. For one cup, you'll need about one large wedge. Cut and peel the wedge. Cut into bite-sized cubes and remove the seeds. Fill the measuring cup and set aside.

Wash and peel the beet. Remove the green parts and cut into small pieces. Set aside.

Wash the watercress thoroughly under cold running water and slightly drain. Torn with hands and set aside.

Now, combine pomegranate, watermelon, beets, and watercress in a juicer and process until well juiced.

Transfer to a serving glass and serve immediately.

Nutrition information per serving: Kcal: 131, Protein: 4.5g, Carbs: 36.1g, Fats: 1.4g

33.   Pepper Kale Juice

Ingredients:

2 medium-sized bell peppers, chopped

1 cup of fresh kale, chopped

1 large radish, trimmed

1 cup of avocado, cubed

1 cup of cucumber, sliced

Preparation:

Wash the bell peppers and cut lengthwise in half. Remove the seeds and cut into small pieces. Set aside.

Wash the kale under cold running water and slightly drain. Chop into small pieces and set aside.

Peel and wash the radish. Trim off the green parts and cut into small pieces. Set aside.

Peel the avocado and cut in half. Remove the pit and cut into small cubes. Fill the measuring cup and reserve the rest for later.

Wash the cucumber and cut into thin slices. Fill the measuring cup and reserve the rest for later. Set aside.

Now, combine bell peppers, kale, radish, avocado, and cucumber in a juicer and process until well juiced. Transfer to a serving glass and serve immediately.

Nutrition information per serving: Kcal: 131, Protein: 4.5g, Carbs: 36.1g, Fats: 1.4g

34.   Apricot Cherry Juice

Ingredients:

1 cup of apricots, pitted

1 cup of cherries, pitted

1 small ginger slice, peeled

1 oz. of coconut water

Preparation:

Wash the apricots and cut in half. Remove the pits and cut into small pieces. Fill the measuring cup and set aside.

Wash the cherries and remove the stems, if any. Cut each in half and remove the pits. Fill the measuring cup and set aside.

Peel the ginger slice and set aside.

Now, combine apricots, cherries, and ginger in a juicer and process until well juiced. Transfer to a serving glass and stir in the coconut water.

Refrigerate for 10 minutes before serving.

Enjoy!

Nutrition information per serving: Kcal: 149, Protein: 3.8g, Carbs: 40.8g, Fats: 0.9g

35.   Plum Cabbage Juice

Ingredients:

4 whole plums, chopped

1 cup of purple cabbage, shredded

1 cup of blueberries

1 whole lime, peeled

Preparation:

Wash the plums and cut each in half. Remove the pits and cut into bite-sized pieces. Set aside.

Wash the cabbage thoroughly and shred it. Fill the measuring cup and set aside. Reserve the rest for some other recipe.

Wash the blueberries and slightly drain. Set aside.

Peel the lime and cut lengthwise in half. Set aside.

Now, combine plums, cabbage, blueberries, and lime in a juicer and process until well juiced. Transfer to a serving glass and add some ice before serving.

Enjoy!

Nutrition information per serving: Kcal: 204, Protein: 4.4g, Carbs: 61.8g, Fats: 1.4g

36.   Papaya Orange Juice

Ingredients:

1 cup of papaya, peeled

1 large orange, wedged

1 whole lime, peeled

1 cup of fresh mint, torn

2 oz. of coconut water

1 tbsp. of liquid honey

Preparation:

Peel the papaya and cut in half. Scoop out the seeds and cut into small chunks. Set aside.

Peel the orange and divide into wedges. Cut each wedge in half and set aside.

Peel the lime and cut lengthwise in half. Set aside.

Wash the mint thoroughly under cold running water and slightly drain. Torn with hands and set aside.

Now, combine papaya, orange, lime, and mint in a juicer and process until well juiced. Transfer to a serving glass and stir in the coconut water.

Add some ice and serve immediately.

Enjoy!

Nutrition information per serving: Kcal: 200, Protein: 3.6g, Carbs: 44.7g, Fats: 0.9g

37.   Coriander Leek Juice

Ingredients:

1 cup of fresh coriander, chopped

2 whole leeks, chopped

1 cup of turnip greens, chopped

1 cup of sweet potatoes, cubed

1 cup of cucumber, sliced

1 whole lime, peeled

1 cup of spinach, chopped

Preparation:

In a large colander, combine coriander, turnip greens, and spinach. Wash thoroughly under cold running water. Chop all into small pieces and set aside.

Wash the leeks and cut into bite-sized pieces. Set aside.

Peel the sweet potato and cut into small cubes. Fill the measuring cup and reserve the rest for later. Set aside.

Wash the cucumber and cut into thin slices. Fill the measuring cup and reserve the rest for later. Set aside.

Peel the lime and cut lengthwise in half. Set aside.

Now, combine coriander, turnip greens, spinach, leeks, sweet potatoes, and cucumber in a juicer. Process until well juiced.

Transfer to a serving glass and serve immediately.

Nutrition information per serving: Kcal: 264, Protein: 2.2g, Carbs: 72.8g, Fats: 13.9g

38.   Broccoli Zucchini Juice

Ingredients:

1 cup of broccoli, chopped

1 small zucchini, chopped

1 cup of green peas

1 cup of Brussels sprouts

1 cup of cucumber, sliced

1 small ginger slice, peeled

Preparation:

Wash the broccoli and trim off the outer layers. Cut into small pieces and set aside.

Peel the zucchini and cut into bite-sized pieces. Set aside.

Wash the Brussels sprouts and trim off the outer wilted leaves. Cut in half and set aside.

Wash the cucumber and cut into thin slices. Fill the measuring cup and reserve the rest for later. Set aside.

Now, combine broccoli, zucchini, Brussels sprouts, and cucumber in a juicer and process until well juiced. Transfer to a serving glass and serve immediately.

Nutrition information per serving: Kcal: 160, Protein: 15.3g, Carbs: 41.5g, Fats: 1.6g

39.   Avocado Plum Juice

Ingredients:

1 cup of avocado, cubed

2 whole plums, chopped

1 medium-sized apple, cored

1 whole lemon, peeled

¼ tsp of cinnamon, ground

1 tbsp. of coconut water

Preparation:

Peel the avocado and cut in half. Remove the pit and cut into small cubes. Fill the measuring cup and reserve the rest for later.

Wash the plums and cut lengthwise in half. Remove the pits and cut into bite-sized pieces. Set aside.

Wash the apple and cut in half. Remove the pit and cut into small pieces. Set aside.

Peel the lemon and cut into half. Set aside.

Now, combine avocado, plums, apple, and lemon in a juicer and process until juiced. Transfer to a serving glass and stir in the cinnamon and coconut water.

Refrigerate for 15 minutes before serving.

Enjoy!

Nutrition information per serving: Kcal: 341, Protein: 5.3g, Carbs: 56.1g, Fats: 22.8g

40.   Pumpkin Apple Juice

Ingredients:

1 cup of pumpkin, cubed

1 small Granny Smith's apple, cored

1 medium-sized carrot, sliced

1 cup of cucumber, sliced

¼ tsp of cinnamon, ground

¼ tsp of ginger, ground

Preparation:

Cut the pumpkin in half and scoop out the seeds. Wash it and cut one large wedge. Peel it and cut into small cubes. Fill the measuring cup and reserve the rest in the refrigerator.

Wash the apple and cut lengthwise in half. Remove the core and cut into small pieces. Set aside.

Wash and peel the carrot. Cut into thin slices and set aside.

Wash the cucumber and cut into thin slices. Fill the measuring cup and reserve the rest for later.

Now, combine pumpkin, apple, carrot, and cucumber in a juicer and process until juiced. Transfer to a serving glass and stir in the cinnamon and ginger.

Refrigerate for 10 minutes before serving.

Nutritional information per serving: Kcal: 121, Protein: 2.7g, Carbs: 34.8g, Fats: 0.6g

41.   Peach Lime Juice

Ingredients:

2 large peaches, pitted

1 whole lime, peeled

1 cup of apricots, sliced

1 large banana, peeled

Preparation:

Wash the peaches and cut in half. Remove the pits and cut each half into bite-sized pieces. Set aside.

Peel the lime and roughly chop it. Make sure to reserve lime juice while cutting.

Wash the apricots and cut in half. Remove the pits and cut into small pieces. Fill the measuring cup and set aside.

Peel the banana and cut into small chunks. Set aside.

Now, combine peaches, lime, apricots, and banana in a juicer and process until juiced. Transfer to a serving glass and add some crushed ice before serving.

Enjoy!

Nutritional information per serving: Kcal: 299, Protein: 7.2g, Carbs: 86.5g, Fats: 2g

42.   Artichoke Spinach Juice

Ingredients:

1 medium-sized artichoke, chopped

1 cup of fresh spinach, chopped

1 cup of green beans, chopped

1 small green bell pepper, sliced

1 small ginger knob, peeled and sliced

Preparation:

Trim off the outer leaves of the artichoke using a sharp paring knife. Wash it and cut into bite-sized pieces. Set aside.

Using a colander, rinse the spinach thoroughly under cold running water. Chop into small pieces and set aside.

Place the beans in a deep pot. Add 1 cup of water and bring it to a boil. Cook for 5 minutes and remove from the heat. Set aside to cool completely.

Wash the bell pepper and cut in half. Remove the seeds and stem. Cut into small rings and set aside.

Peel the ginger knob and chop it into small pieces. Set aside.

Now, combine artichoke, spinach, green beans, bell pepper, and ginger in a juicer and process until juiced. Transfer to a serving glass and refrigerate for 10 minutes before serving.

Nutritional information per serving: Kcal: 95, Protein: 11.9g, Carbs: 29.4g, Fats: 1.3g

43.   Orange Pear Juice

Ingredients:

1 medium-sized orange, peeled

1 medium-sized pear, chopped

1 whole plum, pitted

1 whole lemon, peeled

1 oz. of water

Preparation:

Peel the orange and divide into wedges. Cut each wedge in half and set aside.

Wash the pear and cut in half. Remove the core and chop into small pieces. Set aside.

Wash the plum and cut in half. Remove the pit and cut in small pieces.

Peel the lemon and cut into quarters. Set aside.

Now, combine orange, pear, plum, and lemon in a juicer and process until juiced. Transfer to a serving glass and stir in the water.

You can add a pinch of minced mint for some extra smooth flavor, but it's optional.

Add some crushed ice and serve immediately.

Nutritional information per serving: Kcal: 166, Protein: 2.9g, Carbs: 55.4g, Fats: 0.8g

44. Raspberry Carrot Juice

Ingredients:

1 cup of raspberries

2 large carrots, peeled and chopped

1 large orange, wedged

¼ tsp of ginger, ground

1 tbsp. of liquid honey

Preparation:

Using a colander, rinse the raspberries under cold running water and drain. Set aside.

Wash the carrots and peel them. Cut into small chunks and set aside.

Peel the orange and divide into wedges. Set aside.

Now, combine raspberries, carrots, and orange in a juicer and process until well juiced. Transfer to a serving glass and stir in the ginger and honey.

Refrigerate for 15 minutes before serving.

ADDITIONAL TITLES FROM THIS AUTHOR

70 Effective Meal Recipes to Prevent and Solve Being Overweight: Burn Fat Fast by Using Proper Dieting and Smart Nutrition

By

Joe Correa CSN

48 Acne Solving Meal Recipes: The Fast and Natural Path to Fixing Your Acne Problems in Less Than 10 Days!

By

Joe Correa CSN

41 Alzheimer's Preventing Meal Recipes: Reduce or Eliminate Your Alzheimer's Condition in 30 Days or Less!

By

Joe Correa CSN

70 Effective Breast Cancer Meal Recipes: Prevent and Fight Breast Cancer with Smart Nutrition and Powerful Foods

By

Joe Correa CSN

www.ingramcontent.com/pod-product-compliance
Lightning Source LLC
Chambersburg PA
CBHW030250030426
42336CB00009B/328